*T*his book is a record of

the love and good wishes I've received

while I've been getting well.

name _____

_____

place _____

_____

dates _____

_____

THE GET WELL BOOK

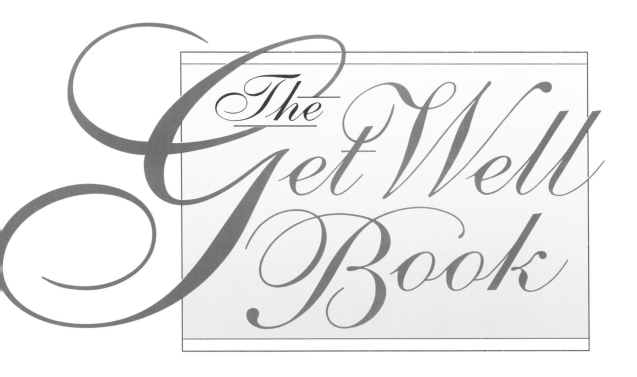

The Get Well Book

Created, designed, and illustrated by

LEONARD TODD

VIKING STUDIO BOOKS

AUTHOR'S NOTE

Several years ago, my mother was in the hospital for an operation. Many of her friends came to visit or sent flowers and cards. She and my father and I tried to keep a record of these expressions of love, but our notes on stray slips of paper were easily misplaced.

Since designing books is part of my professional life, I realized that a single volume for keeping such records would be a great help to those who are sick. It could combine a visitors register, a listing of doctors and nurses, space for noting flowers received, and a journal for charting progress toward health.

My mother recovered from her illness and helped me create this book. She wrote the poem that appears at the end of the last section. It's also a good one to start with:

> I shall look to the East
> Where the sun comes up
> And reach for things from afar.
> Some people ride in subways—
> I much prefer a star!

THE GET WELL BOOK

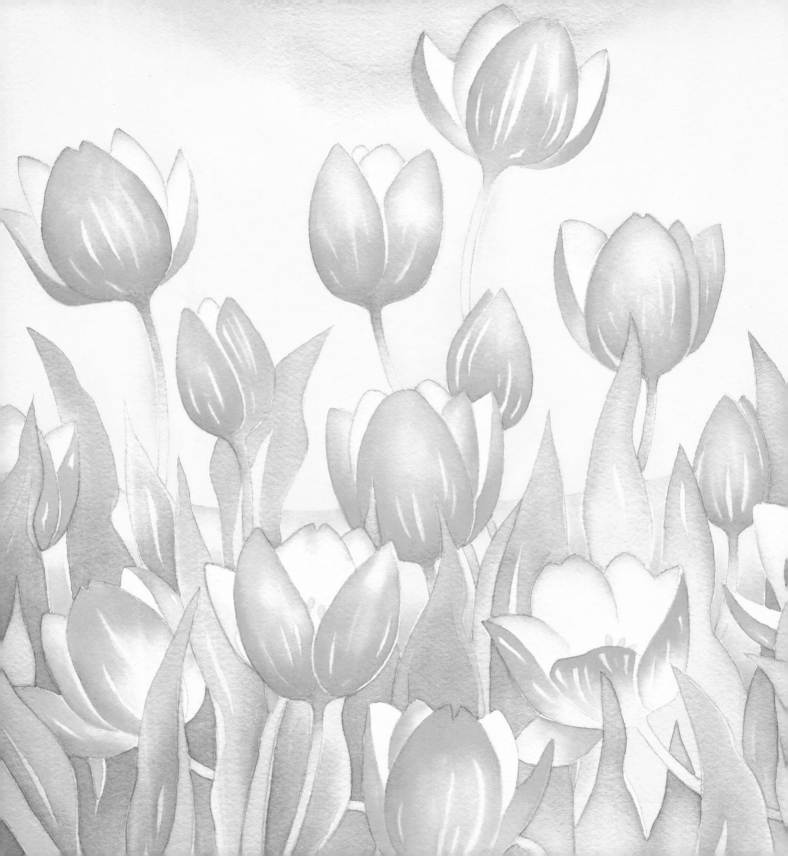

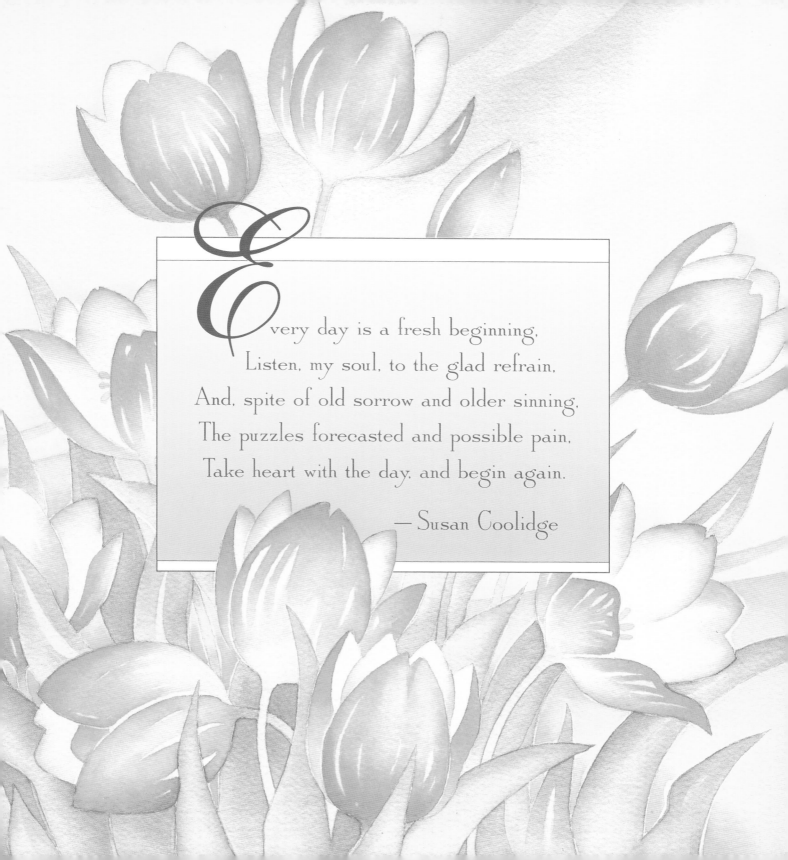

Every day is a fresh beginning,
Listen, my soul, to the glad refrain,
And, spite of old sorrow and older sinning,
The puzzles forecasted and possible pain,
Take heart with the day, and begin again.

— Susan Coolidge

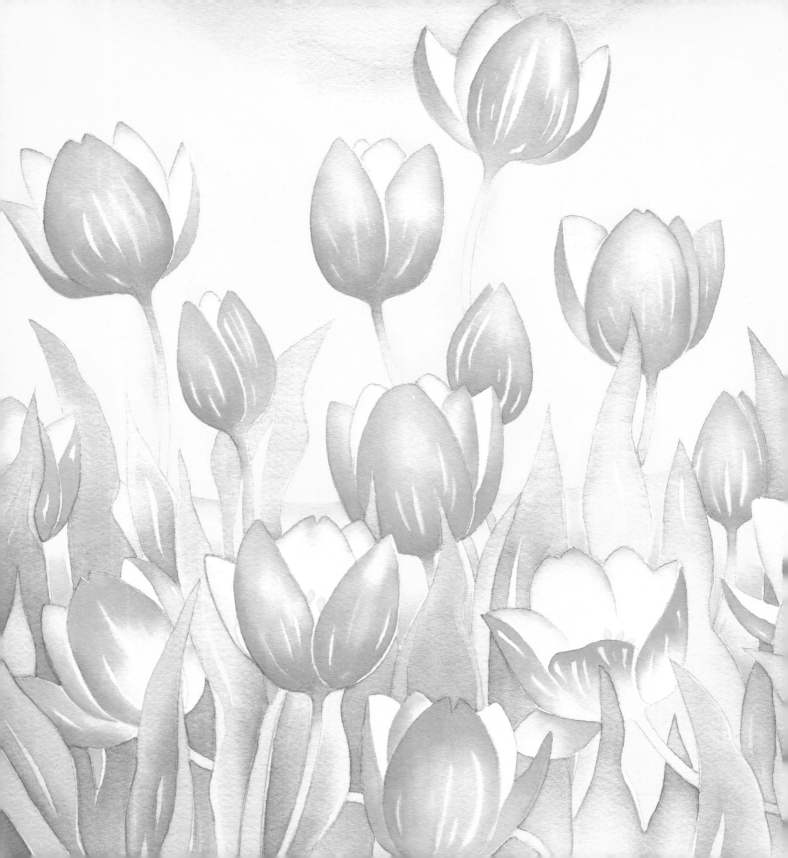

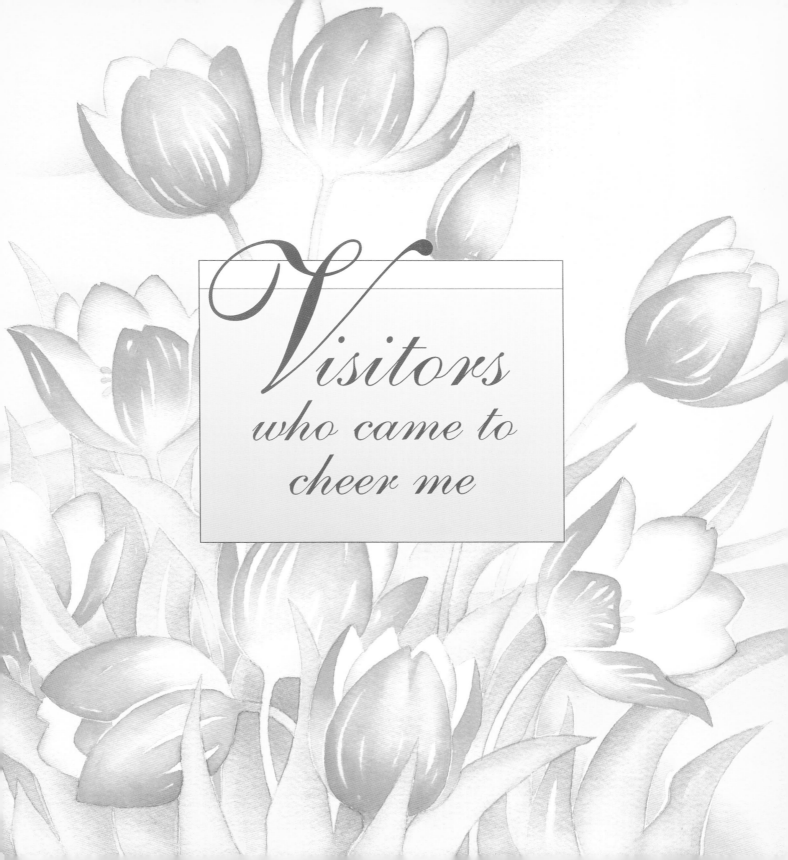

Visitors
who came to
cheer me

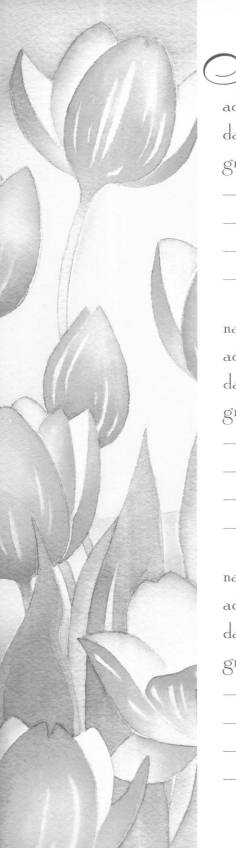

$\mathcal{N}$ame _____

address _____

date _____

greeting _____

_____

_____

_____

_____

_____

name _____

address _____

date _____

greeting _____

_____

_____

_____

_____

name _____

address _____

date _____

greeting _____

_____

_____

_____

_____

name _____

address _____

date _____

greeting _____

_____

_____

_____

_____

name _____

address _____

date _____

greeting _____

_____

_____

_____

_____

name _____

address _____

date _____

greeting _____

_____

_____

_____

Visitors

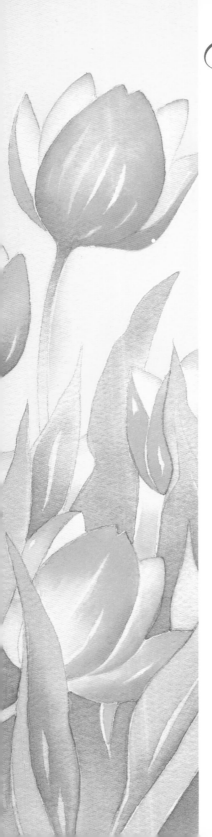

Name _____

address _____

date _____

greeting _____

_____

_____

_____

_____

name _____

address _____

date _____

greeting _____

_____

_____

_____

_____

name _____

address _____

date _____

greeting _____

_____

_____

_____

_____

name

address

date

greeting

name

address

date

greeting

name

address

date

greeting

Visitors

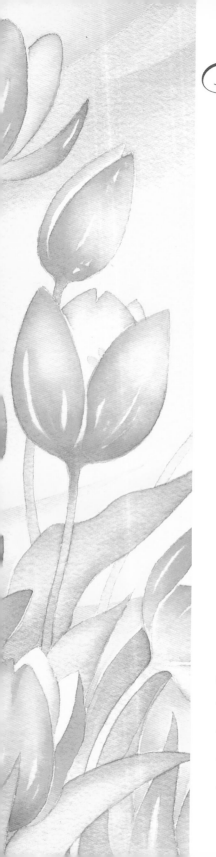

$\mathcal{N}$ame _____

address _____

date _____

greeting _____

_____

_____

_____

_____

name _____

address _____

date _____

greeting _____

_____

_____

_____

_____

name _____

address _____

date _____

greeting _____

_____

_____

_____

_____

name _____

address _____

date _____

greeting _____

_____

_____

_____

_____

name _____

address _____

date _____

greeting _____

_____

_____

_____

_____

name _____

address _____

date _____

greeting _____

_____

_____

_____

_____

Visitors

*N*ame _____

address _____

date _____

greeting _____

_____

_____

_____

_____

_____

name _____

address _____

date _____

greeting _____

_____

_____

_____

_____

name _____

address _____

date _____

greeting _____

_____

_____

_____

_____

name _____

address _____

date _____

greeting _____

_____

_____

_____

_____

name _____

address _____

date _____

greeting _____

_____

_____

_____

name _____

address _____

date _____

greeting _____

_____

_____

_____

Visitors

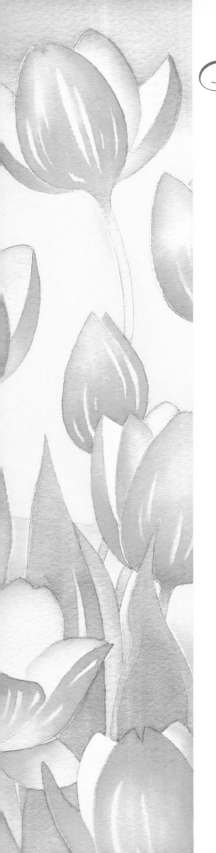

$\mathcal{N}$ame _____

address _____

date _____

greeting _____

_____

_____

_____

_____

name _____

address _____

date _____

greeting _____

_____

_____

_____

_____

name _____

address _____

date _____

greeting _____

_____

_____

_____

_____

name _____

address _____

date _____

greeting _____

_____

_____

_____

_____

name _____

address _____

date _____

greeting _____

_____

_____

_____

_____

name _____

address _____

date _____

greeting _____

_____

_____

_____

_____

Visitors

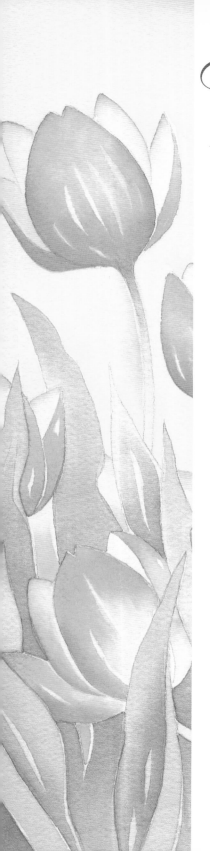

$\mathcal{N}$ame _____

address _____

date _____

greeting _____

_____

_____

_____

_____

name _____

address _____

date _____

greeting _____

_____

_____

_____

_____

name _____

address _____

date _____

greeting _____

_____

_____

_____

_____

name

address

date

greeting

name

address

date

greeting

name

address

date

greeting

Visitors

*N*ame _____

address _____

date _____

greeting _____

_____

_____

_____

_____

name _____

address _____

date _____

greeting _____

_____

_____

_____

_____

name _____

address _____

date _____

greeting _____

_____

_____

_____

_____

name _____

address _____

date _____

greeting _____

_____

_____

_____

_____

name _____

address _____

date _____

greeting _____

_____

_____

_____

_____

name _____

address _____

date _____

greeting _____

_____

_____

_____

_____

Visitors

Name _____

address _____

date _____

greeting _____

_____

_____

_____

_____

name _____

address _____

date _____

greeting _____

_____

_____

_____

_____

name _____

address _____

date _____

greeting _____

_____

_____

_____

_____

name _____

address _____

date _____

greeting _____

_____

_____

_____

_____

_____

name _____

address _____

date _____

greeting _____

_____

_____

_____

_____

_____

name _____

address _____

date _____

greeting _____

_____

_____

_____

_____

_____

Visitors

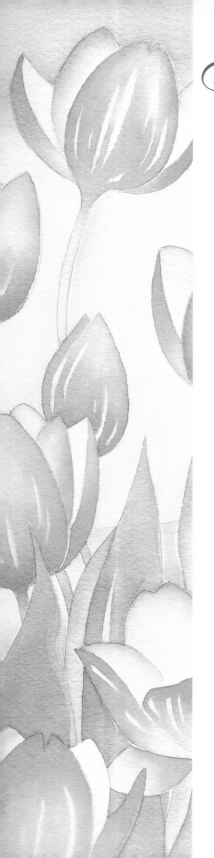

$\mathcal{N}$ame _____

address _____

date _____

greeting _____

_____

_____

_____

_____

name _____

address _____

date _____

greeting _____

_____

_____

_____

_____

name _____

address _____

date _____

greeting _____

_____

_____

_____

_____

name _____

address _____

date _____

greeting _____

_____

_____

_____

_____

name _____

address _____

date _____

greeting _____

_____

_____

_____

_____

name _____

address _____

date _____

greeting _____

_____

_____

_____

Visitors

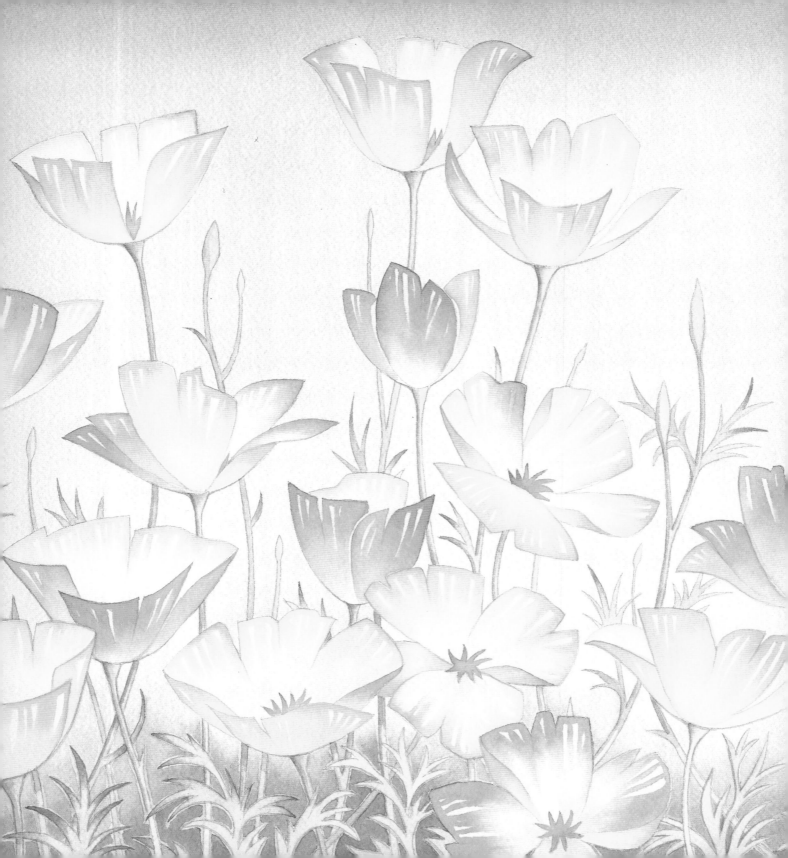

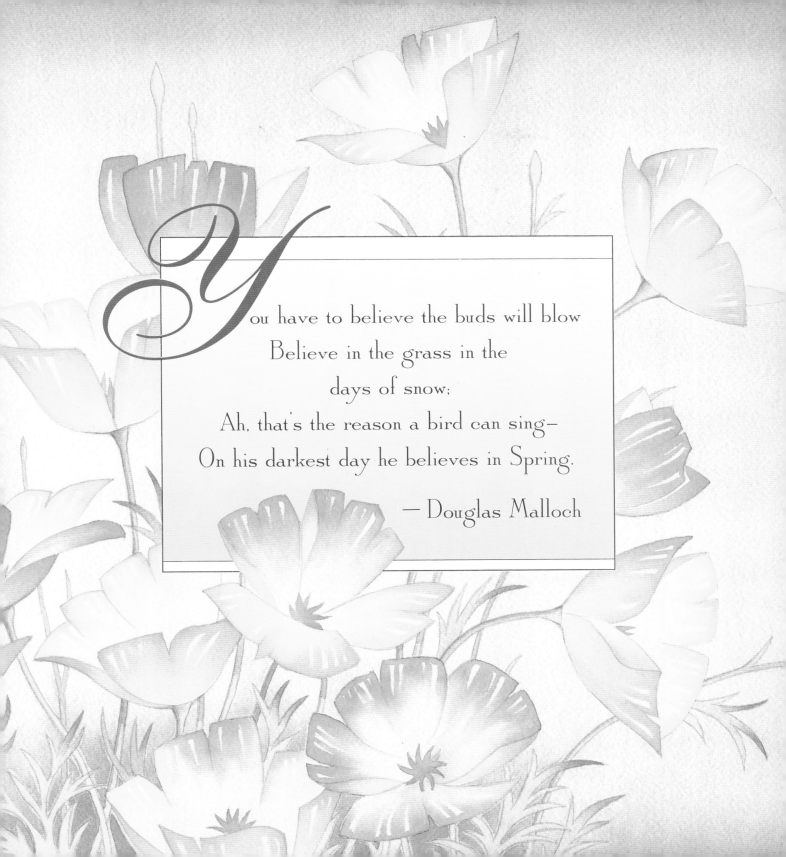

You have to believe the buds will blow
Believe in the grass in the
days of snow;
Ah, that's the reason a bird can sing—
On his darkest day he believes in Spring.

— Douglas Malloch

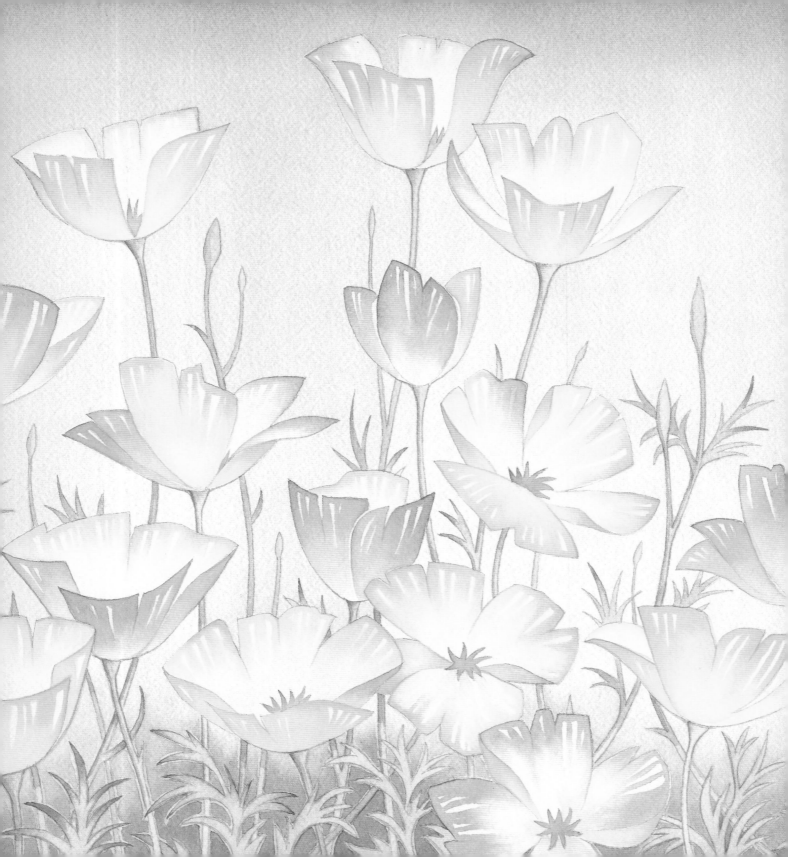

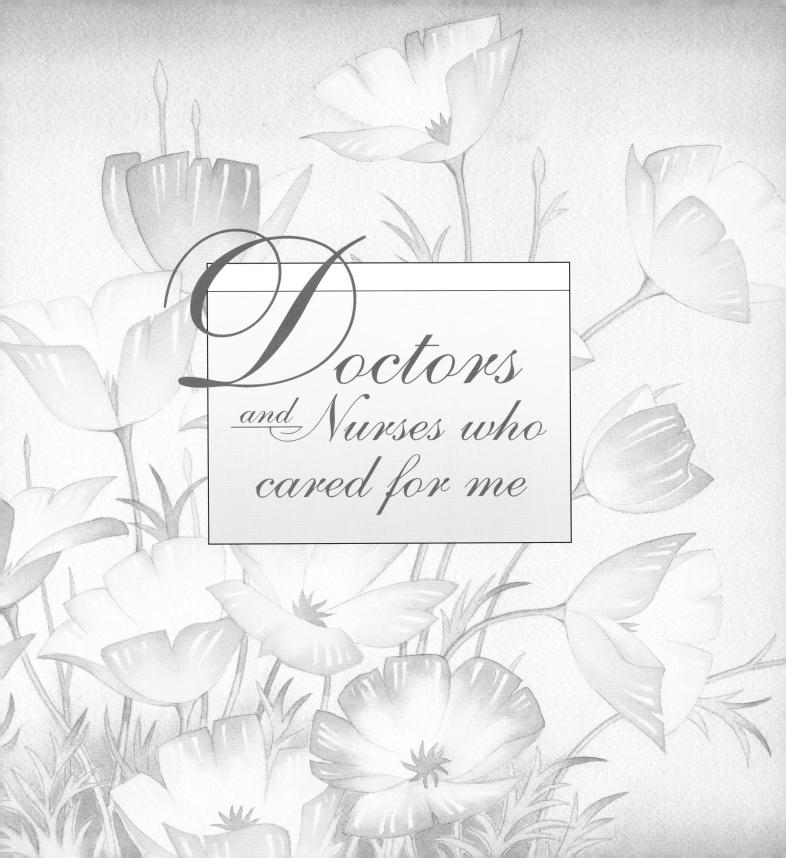

Doctors and Nurses who cared for me

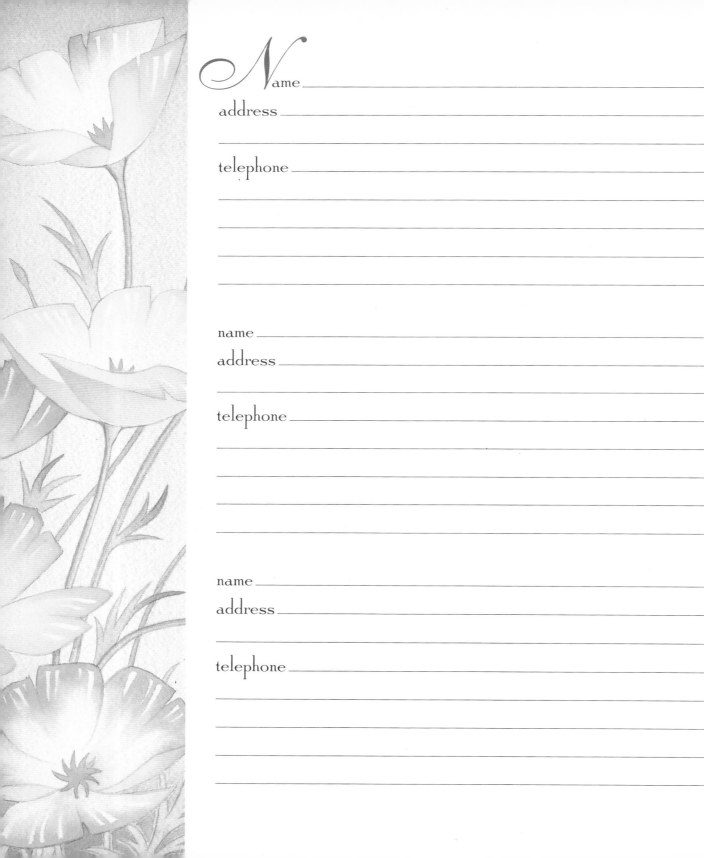

$\mathcal{N}$ame _____

address _____

_____

telephone _____

_____

_____

_____

_____

name _____

address _____

_____

telephone _____

_____

_____

_____

_____

name _____

address _____

_____

telephone _____

_____

_____

_____

_____

name _____

address _____

_____

telephone _____

_____

_____

_____

name _____

address _____

_____

telephone _____

_____

_____

_____

name _____

address _____

_____

telephone _____

_____

_____

_____

Doctors and Nurses

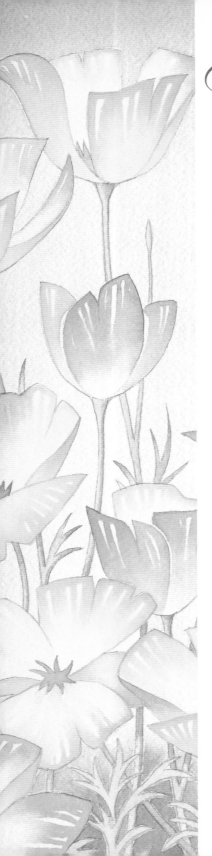

*N*ame _____

address _____

_____

telephone _____

_____

_____

_____

_____

name _____

address _____

_____

telephone _____

_____

_____

_____

_____

name _____

address _____

_____

telephone _____

_____

_____

_____

name _____

address _____

_____

telephone _____

_____

_____

_____

name _____

address _____

_____

telephone _____

_____

_____

_____

name _____

address _____

_____

telephone _____

_____

_____

_____

Doctors and Nurses

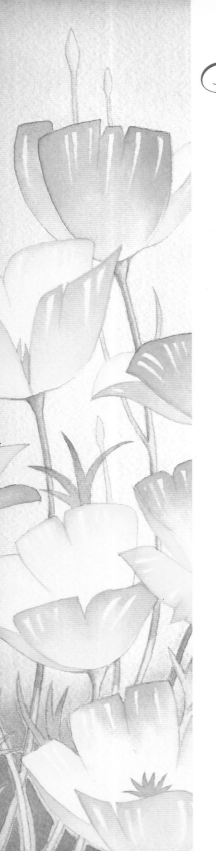

$\mathcal{N}$ame _____

address _____

_____

telephone _____

_____

_____

_____

_____

name _____

address _____

telephone _____

_____

_____

_____

_____

name _____

address _____

telephone _____

_____

_____

_____

name

address

telephone

name

address

telephone

name

address

telephone

Doctors and Nurses

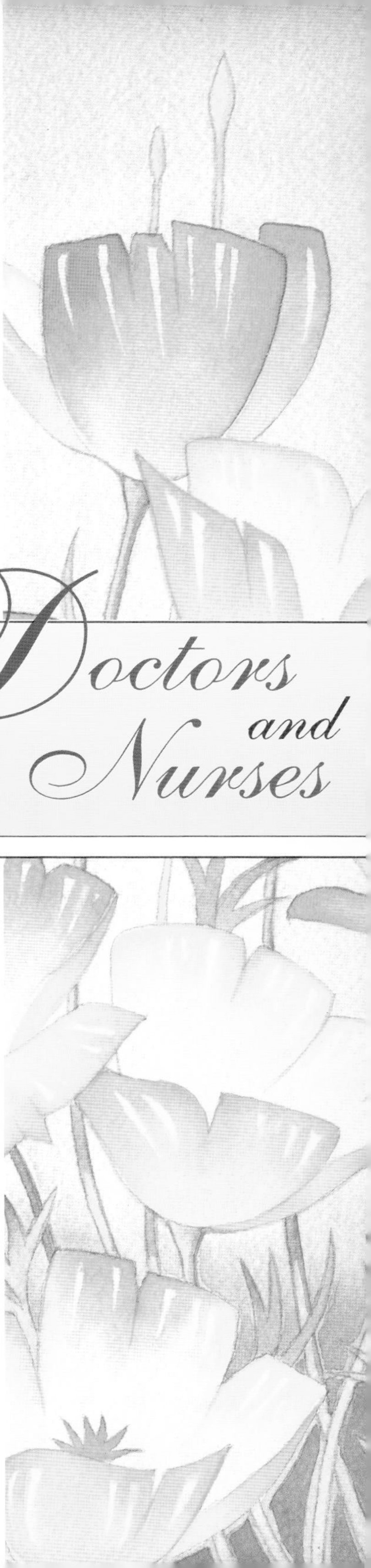

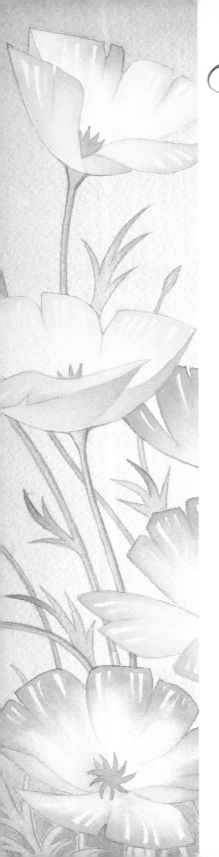

*N*ame _____

address _____

_____

telephone _____

_____

_____

_____

_____

name _____

address _____

_____

telephone _____

_____

_____

_____

_____

name _____

address _____

_____

telephone _____

_____

_____

_____

name _____

address _____

_____

telephone _____

_____

_____

_____

name _____

address _____

_____

telephone _____

_____

_____

_____

name _____

address _____

_____

telephone _____

_____

_____

_____

Doctors and Nurses

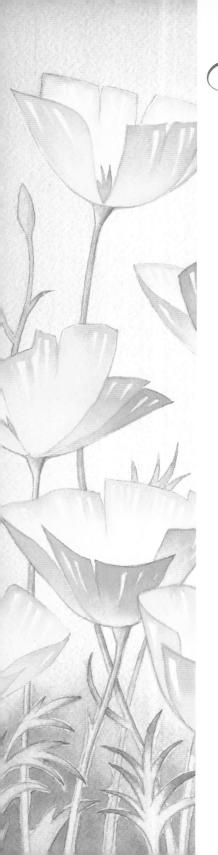

$\mathcal{N}$ame _____

address _____

_____

telephone _____

_____

_____

_____

_____

name _____

address _____

telephone _____

_____

_____

_____

_____

name _____

address _____

telephone _____

_____

_____

_____

name _____

address _____

_____

telephone _____

_____

_____

_____

name _____

address _____

_____

telephone _____

_____

_____

_____

name _____

address _____

_____

telephone _____

_____

_____

_____

Doctors and Nurses

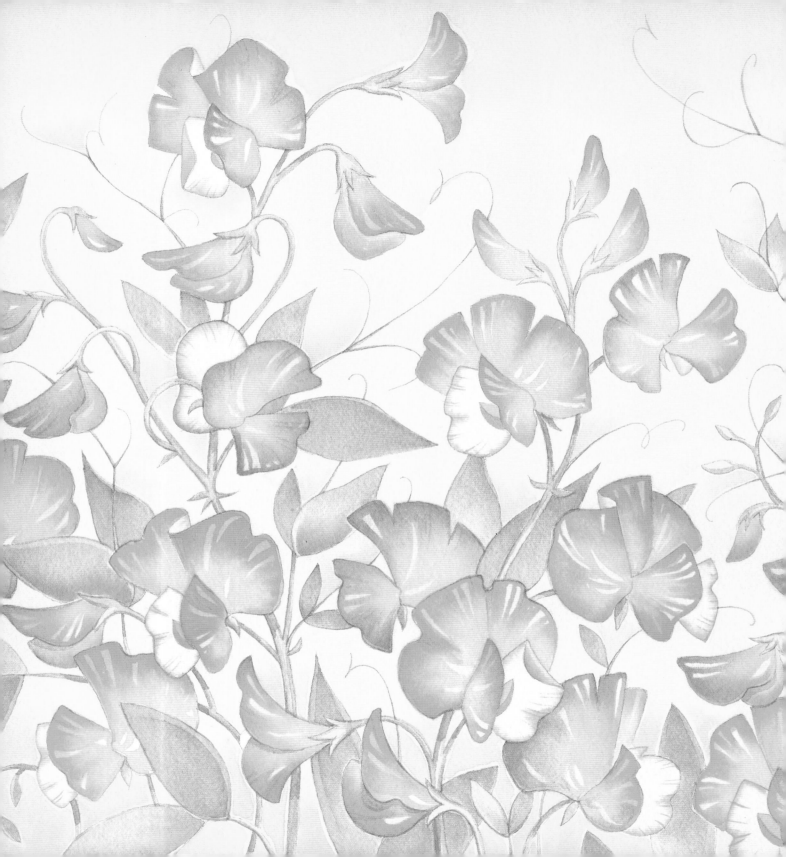

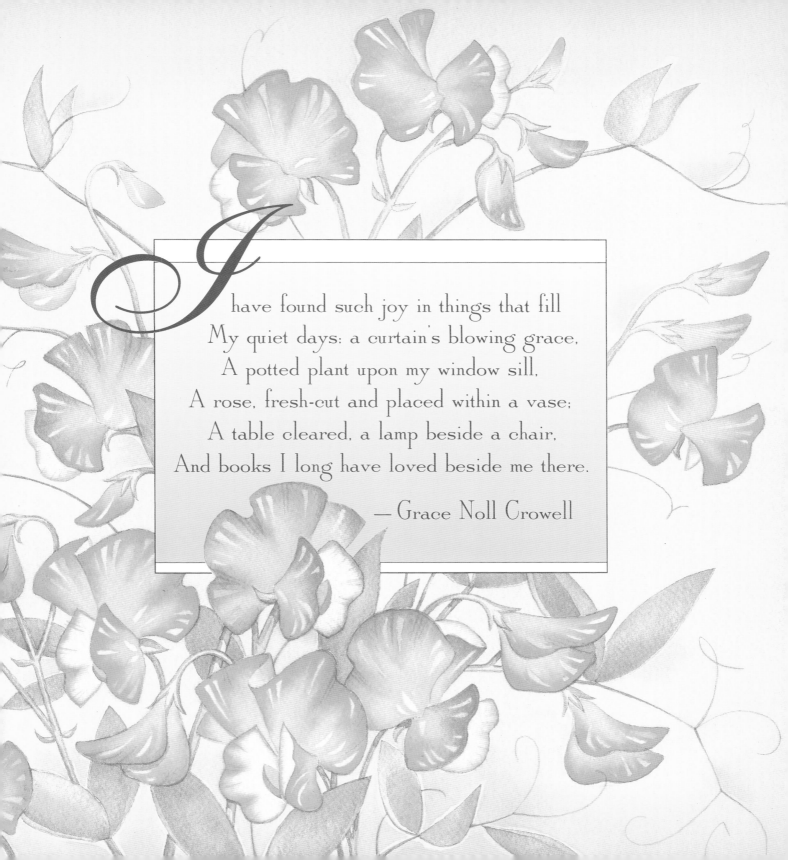

I have found such joy in things that fill
My quiet days: a curtain's blowing grace,
A potted plant upon my window sill,
A rose, fresh-cut and placed within a vase;
A table cleared, a lamp beside a chair,
And books I long have loved beside me there.

— Grace Noll Crowell

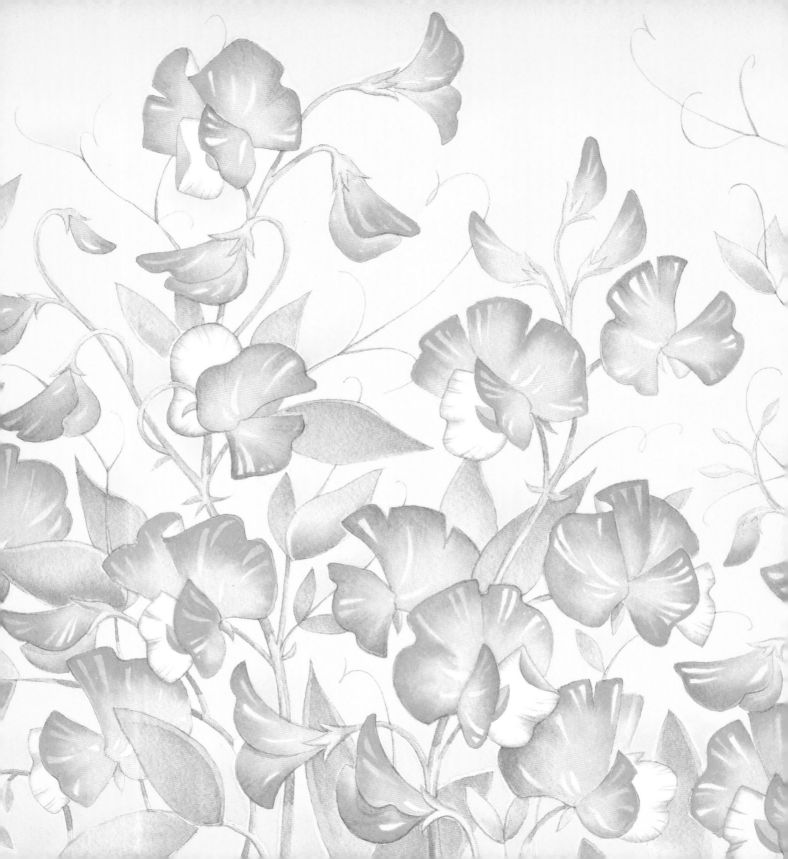

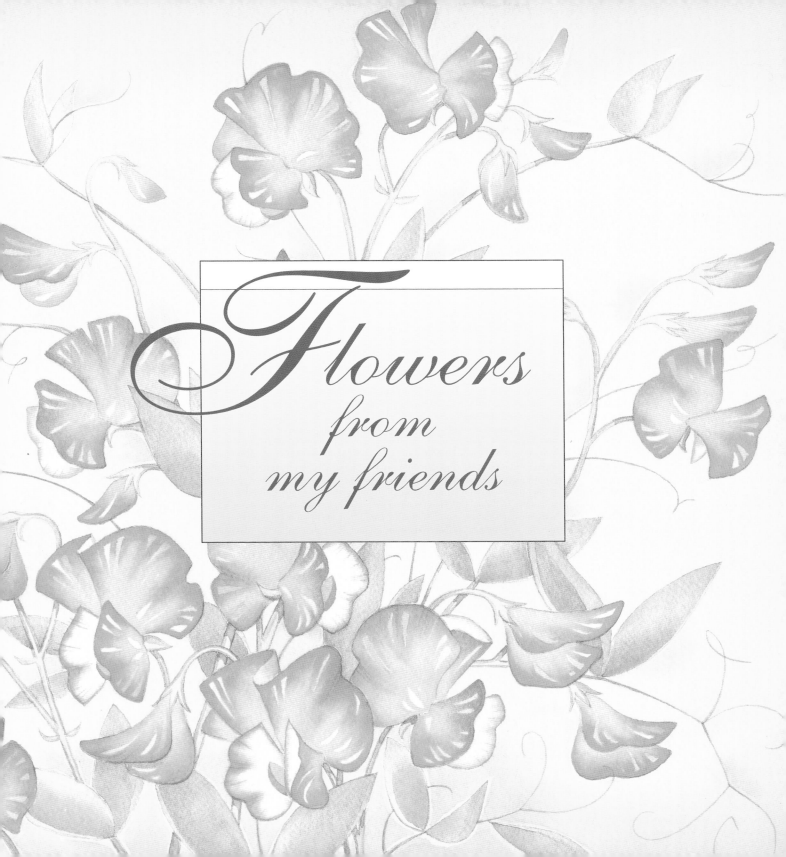

Flowers
from
my friends

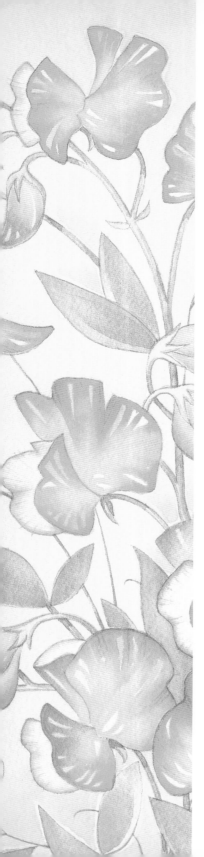

*D*escription _____

name of giver _____

address _____

_____

_____ thank-you note ☐

description _____

name of giver _____

address _____

_____ thank-you note ☐

description _____

name of giver _____

address _____

_____ thank-you note ☐

description _____

name of giver _____

address _____

_____ thank-you note ☐

description _____

name of giver _____

address _____

_____

_____ thank-you note ☐

description _____

name of giver _____

address _____

_____

_____ thank-you note ☐

description _____

name of giver _____

address _____

_____ thank-you note ☐

description _____

name of giver _____

address _____

_____ thank-you note ☐

description _____

name of giver _____

address _____

_____ thank-you note ☐

description _____

name of giver _____

address _____

_____ thank-you note ☐

*Flowers
and Gifts*

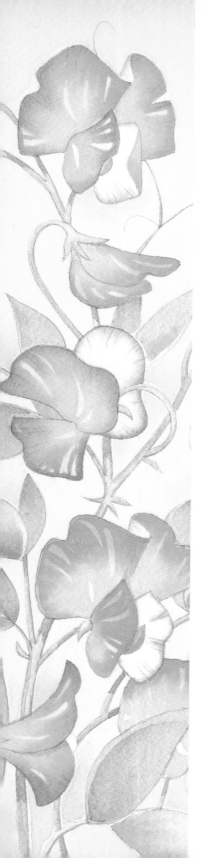

$\mathcal{D}$escription _____

name of giver _____

address _____

_____

_____ thank-you note ☐

description _____

name of giver _____

address _____

_____ thank-you note ☐

description _____

name of giver _____

address _____

_____ thank-you note ☐

description _____

name of giver _____

address _____

_____ thank-you note ☐

description _____

name of giver _____

address _____

_____ thank-you note ☐

description _____

name of giver _____

address _____

_____

_____ thank-you note ☐

description _____

name of giver _____

address _____

_____ thank-you note ☐

description _____

name of giver _____

address _____

_____ thank-you note ☐

description _____

name of giver _____

address _____

_____ thank-you note ☐

description _____

name of giver _____

address _____

_____ thank-you note ☐

Flowers and Gifts

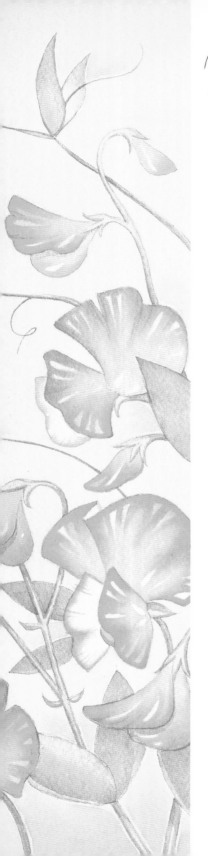

$\mathcal{D}$escription _____

name of giver _____

address _____

_____

_____ thank-you note ☐

description _____

name of giver _____

address _____

_____ thank-you note ☐

description _____

name of giver _____

address _____

_____ thank-you note ☐

description _____

name of giver _____

address _____

_____ thank-you note ☐

description _____

name of giver _____

address _____

_____

_____ thank-you note ☐

description _____

name of giver _____

address _____

_____

_____ thank-you note ☐

description _____

name of giver _____

address _____

_____ thank-you note ☐

description _____

name of giver _____

address _____

_____ thank-you note ☐

description _____

name of giver _____

address _____

_____ thank-you note ☐

description _____

name of giver _____

address _____

_____

_____ thank-you note ☐

Flowers
and Gifts

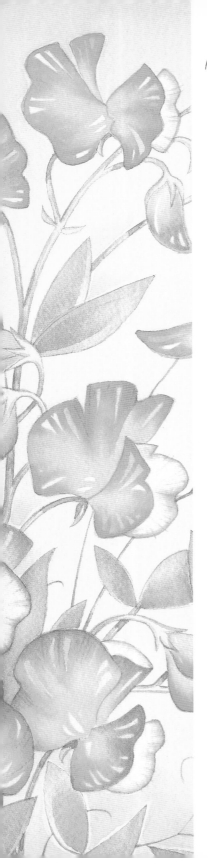

$\mathcal{D}$escription _____

name of giver _____

address _____

_____

_____ thank-you note ☐

description _____

name of giver _____

address _____

_____ thank-you note ☐

description _____

name of giver _____

address _____

_____ thank-you note ☐

description _____

name of giver _____

address _____

_____ thank-you note ☐

description _____

name of giver _____

address _____

_____ thank-you note ☐

description _____

name of giver _____

address _____

_____

_____ thank-you note ☐

description _____

name of giver _____

address _____

_____ thank-you note ☐

description _____

name of giver _____

address _____

_____ thank-you note ☐

description _____

name of giver _____

address _____

_____ thank-you note ☐

description _____

name of giver _____

address _____

_____

_____ thank-you note ☐

Flowers
and Gifts

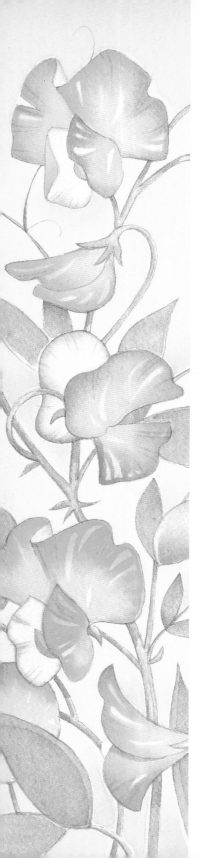

*D*escription _____

name of giver _____

address _____

_____

_____ thank-you note ☐

description _____

name of giver _____

address _____

_____ thank-you note ☐

description _____

name of giver _____

address _____

_____ thank-you note ☐

description _____

name of giver _____

address _____

_____ thank-you note ☐

description _____

name of giver _____

address _____

_____

_____ thank-you note ☐

description _____

name of giver _____

address _____

_____

_____ thank-you note ☐

description _____

name of giver _____

address _____

_____ thank-you note ☐

description _____

name of giver _____

address _____

_____ thank-you note ☐

description _____

name of giver _____

address _____

_____ thank-you note ☐

description _____

name of giver _____

address _____

_____

_____ thank-you note ☐

Flowers
and Gifts

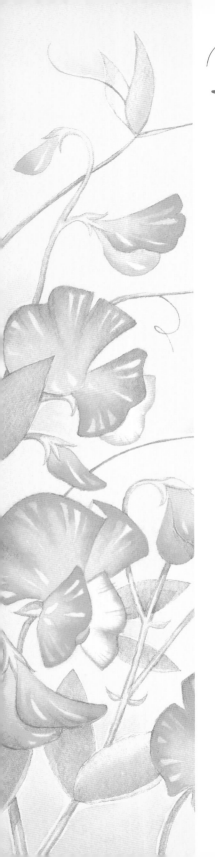

*D*escription _____

name of giver _____

address _____

_____

_____ thank-you note ☐

description _____

name of giver _____

address _____

_____ thank-you note ☐

description _____

name of giver _____

address _____

_____ thank-you note ☐

description _____

name of giver _____

address _____

_____ thank-you note ☐

description _____

name of giver _____

address _____

_____

_____ thank-you note ☐

description _____

name of giver _____

address _____

_____

_____ thank-you note ☐

description _____

name of giver _____

address _____

_____ thank-you note ☐

description _____

name of giver _____

address _____

_____ thank-you note ☐

description _____

name of giver _____

address _____

_____ thank-you note ☐

description _____

name of giver _____

address _____

_____ thank-you note ☐

Flowers and Gifts

$\mathcal{D}$escription _____

name of giver _____

address _____

_____

_____ thank-you note ☐

description _____

name of giver _____

address _____

_____ thank-you note ☐

description _____

name of giver _____

address _____

_____ thank-you note ☐

description _____

name of giver _____

address _____

_____ thank-you note ☐

description _____

name of giver _____

address _____

_____

_____ thank-you note ☐

description _____

name of giver _____

address _____

_____

_____ thank-you note ☐

description _____

name of giver _____

address _____

_____ thank-you note ☐

description _____

name of giver _____

address _____

_____ thank-you note ☐

description _____

name of giver _____

address _____

_____ thank-you note ☐

description _____

name of giver _____

address _____

_____

_____ thank-you note ☐

Flowers and Gifts

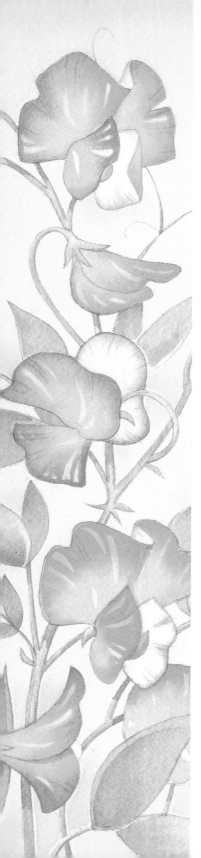

$\mathcal{D}$escription _____

name of giver _____

address _____

_____

_____ thank-you note ☐

description _____

name of giver _____

address _____

_____ thank-you note ☐

description _____

name of giver _____

address _____

_____ thank-you note ☐

description _____

name of giver _____

address _____

_____ thank-you note ☐

description _____

name of giver _____

address _____

_____

_____ thank-you note ☐

description _____

name of giver _____

address _____

_____

_____ thank-you note ☐

description _____

name of giver _____

address _____

_____

_____ thank-you note ☐

description _____

name of giver _____

address _____

_____

_____ thank-you note ☐

description _____

name of giver _____

address _____

_____

_____ thank-you note ☐

description _____

name of giver _____

address _____

_____

_____ thank-you note ☐

Flowers
and Gifts

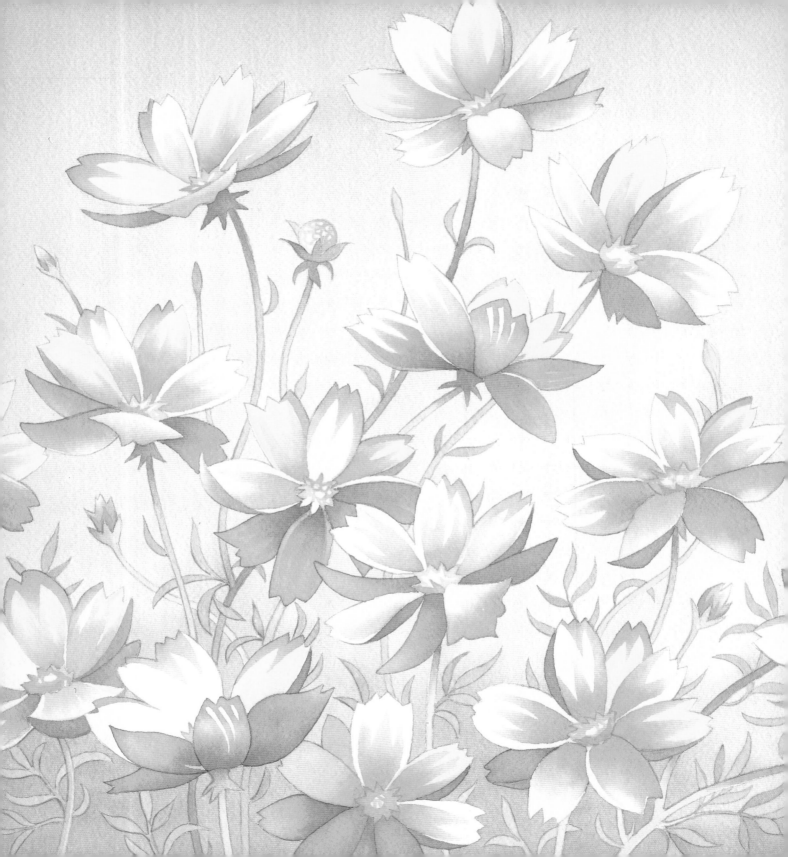

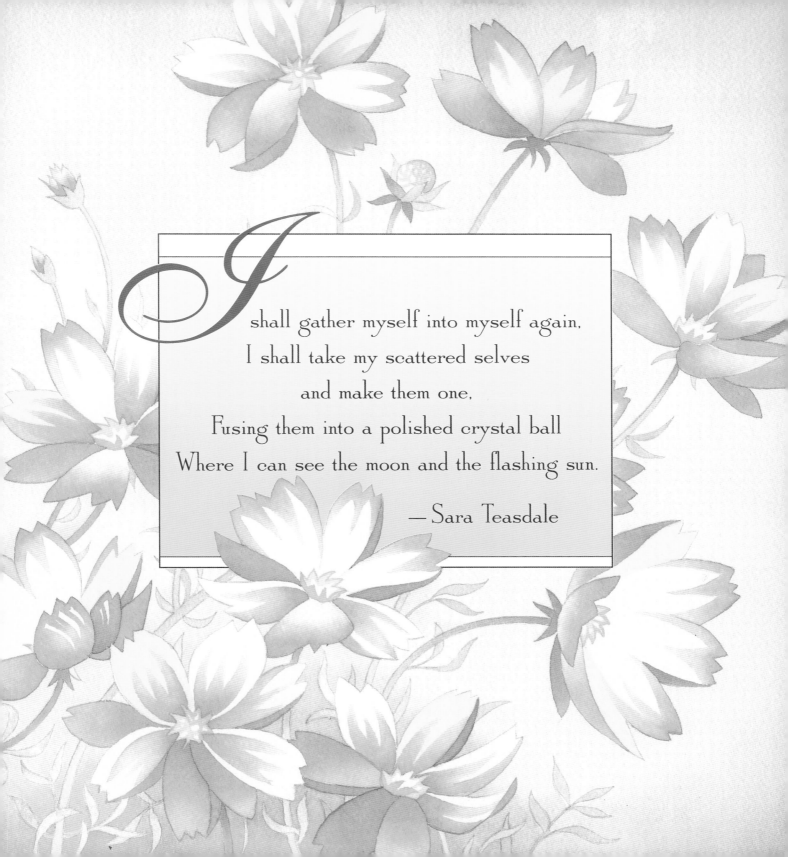

I shall gather myself into myself again,
I shall take my scattered selves
and make them one,
Fusing them into a polished crystal ball
Where I can see the moon and the flashing sun.

— Sara Teasdale

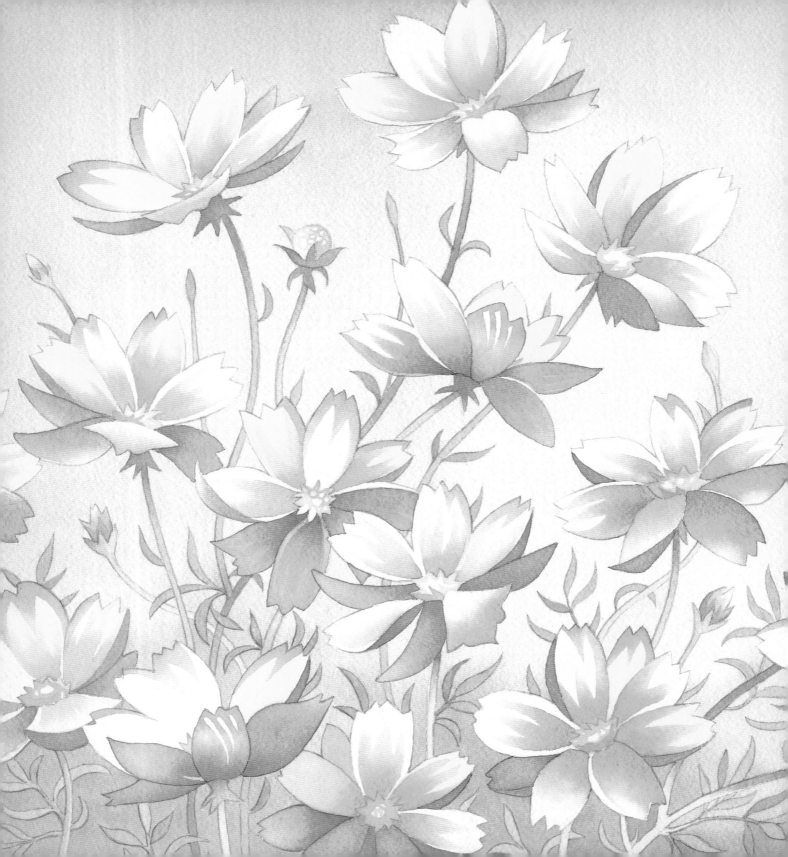

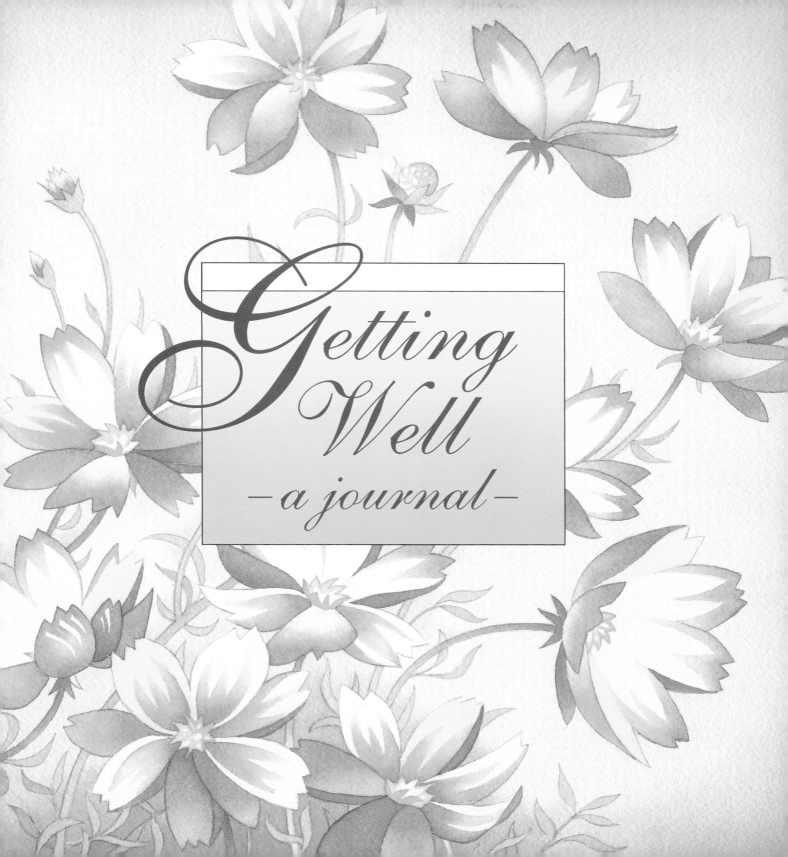

Getting Well
– a journal –

$\mathcal{T}$oday, I am _____ date _____

_____
_____
_____
_____
_____
_____
_____
_____
_____
_____
_____
_____

date _____

Today, I am _____

_____
_____
_____
_____
_____
_____
_____
_____
_____
_____
_____
_____
_____
_____

date _____

Today, I am _____

_____

_____

_____

_____

_____

_____

_____

_____

_____

_____

date _____

Today, I am _____

_____

_____

_____

_____

_____

_____

_____

_____

_____

_____

_____

_____

_____

Getting Well

$\mathcal{T}$oday, I am

date _____

_____
_____
_____
_____
_____
_____
_____
_____
_____
_____
_____

Today, I am

date _____

_____
_____
_____
_____
_____
_____
_____
_____
_____
_____
_____
_____
_____

date _____

Today, I am _____
_____
_____
_____
_____
_____
_____
_____
_____

Getting Well

date _____

Today, I am _____
_____
_____
_____
_____
_____
_____
_____
_____
_____
_____

$\mathcal{T}$oday, I am

date _____

_____
_____
_____
_____
_____
_____
_____
_____
_____

Today, I am

date _____

_____
_____
_____
_____
_____
_____
_____
_____
_____
_____
_____
_____
_____

date _____

Today, I am _____

_____

_____

_____

_____

_____

_____

_____

_____

_____

Getting Well

date _____

Today, I am _____

_____

_____

_____

_____

_____

_____

_____

_____

_____

_____

_____

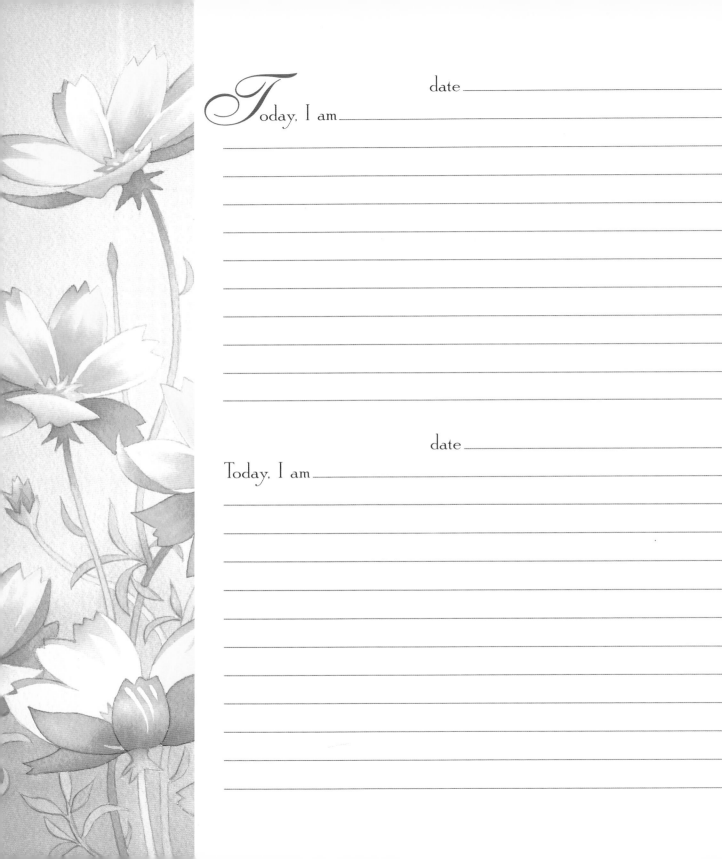

$\mathscr{T}$oday, I am_____

date _____

_____

_____

_____

_____

_____

_____

_____

_____

_____

_____

_____

_____

date _____

Today, I am_____

_____

_____

_____

_____

_____

_____

_____

_____

_____

_____

_____

_____

date _____

Today, I am _____
_____
_____
_____
_____
_____
_____
_____
_____
_____

date _____

Today, I am _____
_____
_____
_____
_____
_____
_____
_____
_____
_____
_____
_____
_____

Getting Well

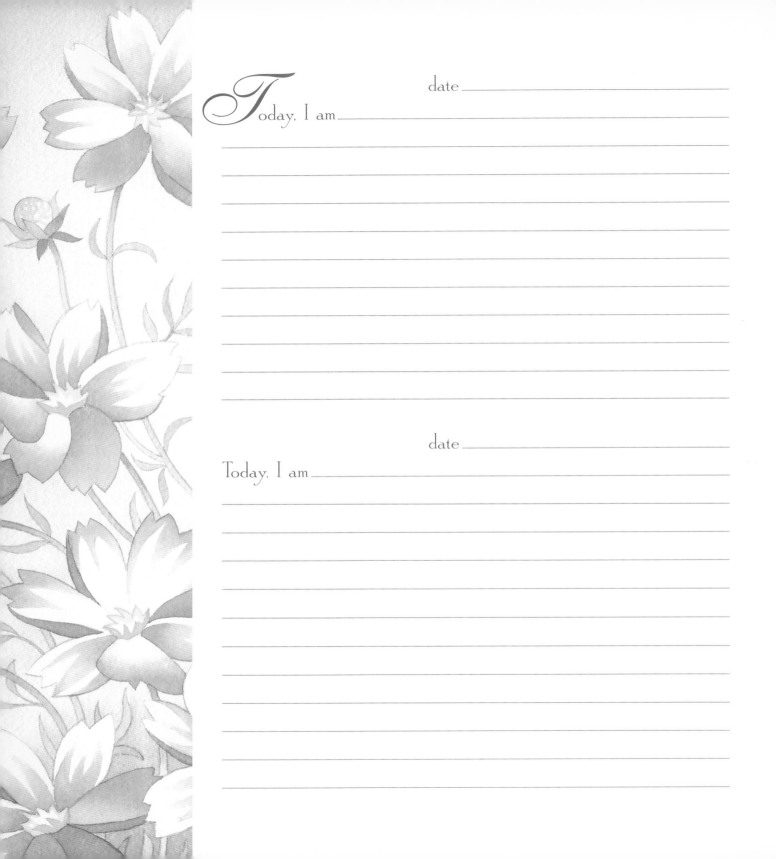

$\mathcal{T}$oday, I am

date

Today, I am

date

date _____

Today, I am _____
_____
_____
_____
_____
_____
_____
_____
_____

date _____

Today, I am _____
_____
_____
_____
_____
_____
_____
_____
_____
_____
_____
_____

Getting Well

$\mathcal{T}$oday, I am

date

Today, I am

date

date _____

Today, I am _____
_____
_____
_____
_____
_____
_____
_____
_____
_____
_____

date _____

Today, I am _____
_____
_____
_____
_____
_____
_____
_____
_____
_____
_____
_____

Getting Well

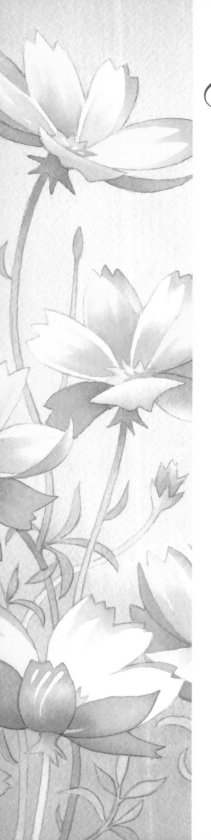

$\mathcal{T}$oday, I am _____

date _____

_____
_____
_____
_____
_____
_____
_____
_____
_____
_____
_____
_____
_____

date _____

Today, I am _____

_____
_____
_____
_____
_____
_____
_____
_____
_____
_____
_____
_____
_____
_____

date _____

Today, I am _____

_____

_____

_____

_____

_____

_____

_____

_____

_____

date _____

Today, I am _____

_____

_____

_____

_____

_____

_____

_____

_____

_____

_____

_____

_____

Getting Well

$\mathcal{T}$oday, I am

date _____

_____
_____
_____
_____
_____
_____
_____
_____
_____
_____

date _____

Today, I am

_____
_____
_____
_____
_____
_____
_____
_____
_____
_____
_____
_____
_____
_____

date _____

Today, I am _____

_____
_____
_____
_____
_____
_____
_____
_____
_____
_____
_____

date _____

Today, I am _____

_____
_____
_____
_____
_____
_____
_____
_____
_____
_____
_____
_____

Getting Well

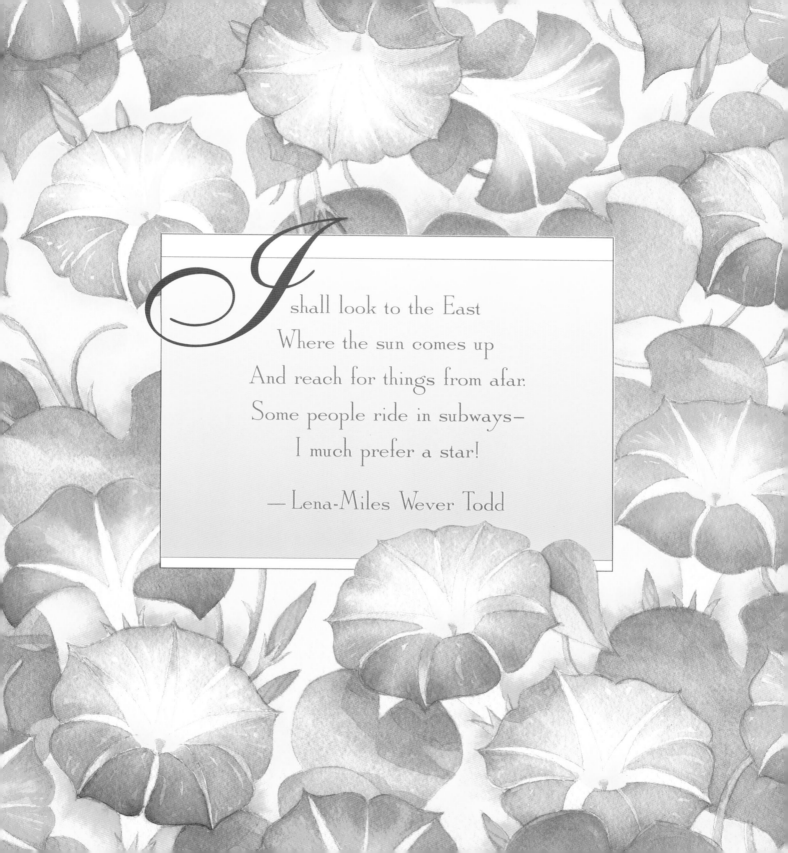

I shall look to the East
Where the sun comes up
And reach for things from afar.
Some people ride in subways—
I much prefer a star!

—Lena-Miles Wever Todd

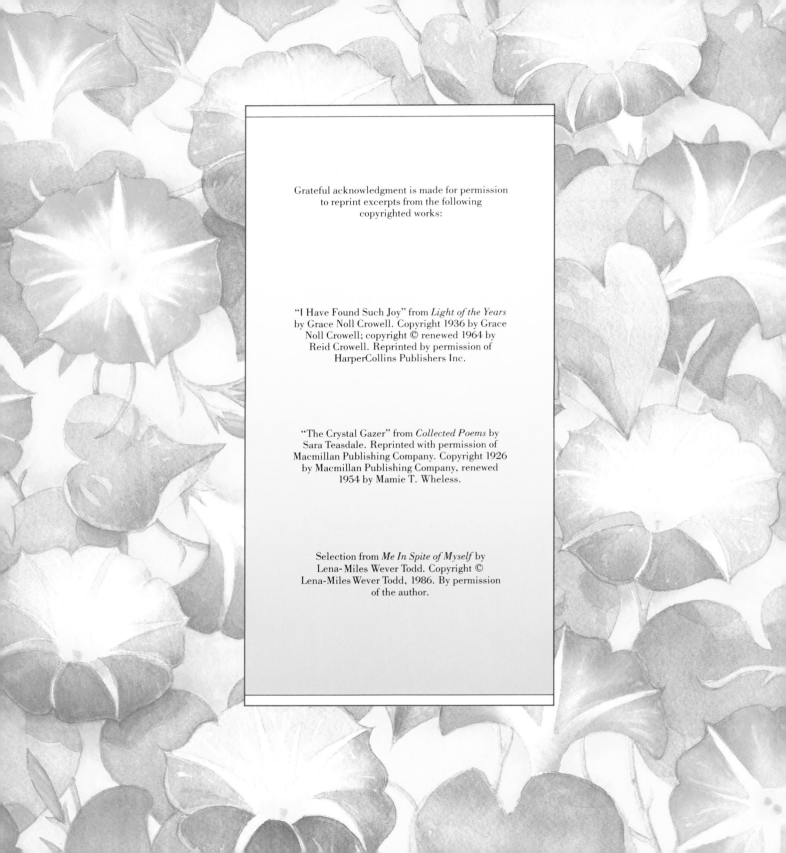

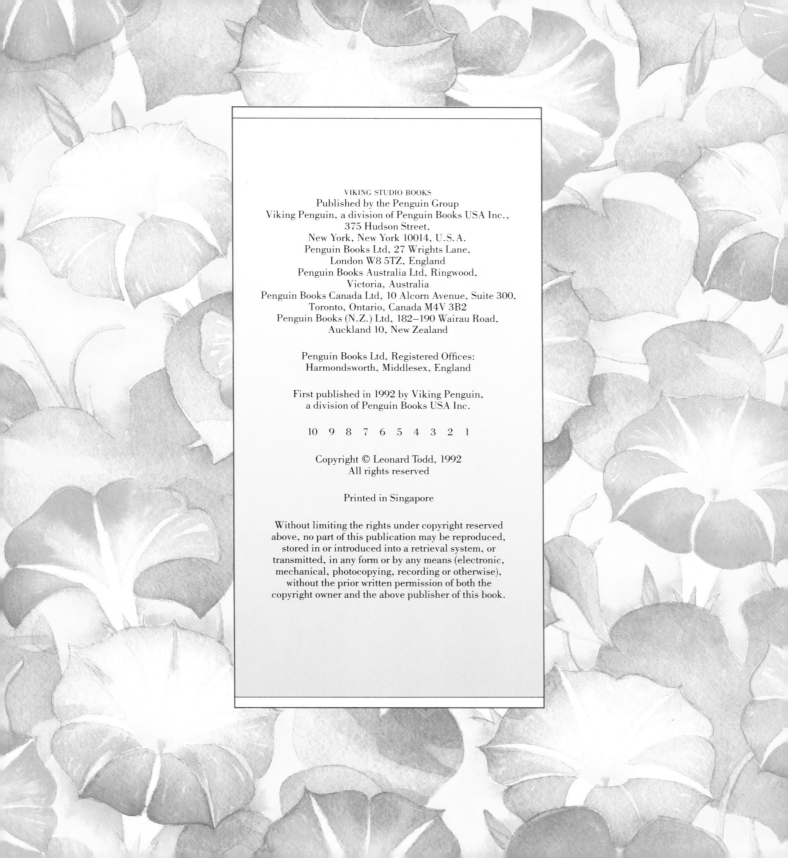

VIKING STUDIO BOOKS
Published by the Penguin Group
Viking Penguin, a division of Penguin Books USA Inc.,
375 Hudson Street,
New York, New York 10014, U.S.A.
Penguin Books Ltd, 27 Wrights Lane,
London W8 5TZ, England
Penguin Books Australia Ltd, Ringwood,
Victoria, Australia
Penguin Books Canada Ltd, 10 Alcorn Avenue, Suite 300,
Toronto, Ontario, Canada M4V 3B2
Penguin Books (N.Z.) Ltd, 182–190 Wairau Road,
Auckland 10, New Zealand

Penguin Books Ltd, Registered Offices:
Harmondsworth, Middlesex, England

First published in 1992 by Viking Penguin,
a division of Penguin Books USA Inc.

10 9 8 7 6 5 4 3 2 1

Copyright © Leonard Todd, 1992
All rights reserved

Printed in Singapore